I0902225

# SO . . . YOU HAVE DECIDED TO BECOME A PHYSICIAN

Professor Linos has eloquently delivered his advice for aspiring physicians. To Dr. Linos' exhortations, I will add my own: Do not measure your own success using someone else's ruler.

To enable a healthy and satisfying profession, we must allow for different definitions of success. We must support an inclusive spectrum of professional choices delivering a diverse set of people, their talents and their interests, and we must not shunt ourselves or others aside when they bristle at our established paradigms. Success cannot be narrowly defined as attending a certain school, or attaining a lofty rank.

We owe it to ourselves, our patients, our trainees, and our families to wisely choose our professional expectations. Dr. Linos' advice will help those interested in medicine to understand the established pathways of education and training, and to position themselves to then chart their own course.

Gerard M. Doherty, M.D.
Moseley Professor of Surgery, Harvard Medical School,
Surgeon-in-Chief,
Brigham Health and Dana-Farber Cancer Institute,
Crowley Family Distinguished Chair,
Department of Surgery, Brigham and Women's Hospital

*So . . . You Have Decided to Become a Physician* by Prof. Dimitrios Linos, an internationally renowned surgeon, is full of insights and pearls from his own extensive experience with the Europe and American systems of medical training and practice. The book emphasizes the best programs and the common pathways, but also discusses the alternatives. It is especially useful for those who are considering advanced medical training in Europe and America. It is an excellent practical guidebook not only for students who want to become physicians, but also for medical students, residents and fellows who are in training and for those who teach them.

Quan-Yang Duh, M.D.
Professor and Chief of Endocrine Surgery,
Department of Surgery,
University of California, San Francisco

An inspirational "must read" for those contemplating or pursuing a career in medicine! Unique is the scope of what is covered: What it means to be a physician, the nuts and bolts of applying to medical school, and understanding specialty training. All delivered with a global perspective. The book is a string of pearls, succinctly and warmly written. The personal reflections on how to balance a successful career with a fulfilling life apply to any profession.

Allan Siperstein, M.D.
Chair of Endocrine Surgery Department,
Cleveland Clinic

So . . . You Have Decided to Become a Physician:
Advice to Aspiring Young Doctors

By Dimitrios Linos

© The Chinese University of Hong Kong 2020

All rights reserved. No part of this publication may be reproduced or transmitted in any form or by any means, electronic or mechanical, including photocopying, recording, or any information storage and retrieval system, without permission in writing from The Chinese University of Hong Kong.

Illustrations by Dimitrios Linos
Cover design by Bianco Tsai

ISBN: 978-988-237-205-4

Published by:
The Chinese University of Hong Kong Press
The Chinese University of Hong Kong
Sha Tin, N.T., Hong Kong
Fax: +852 2603 7355
Email: cup@cuhk.edu.hk
Website: cup.cuhk.edu.hk

Printed in Hong Kong

*So . . .*

# You Have Decided to Become a Physician

Advice to Aspiring Young Doctors

Dimitrios Linos

The Chinese University of Hong Kong Press

# CONTENTS

# FOREWORD

James Y. W. Lau

In 2018, Professor Linos visited The Chinese University of Hong Kong as an external examiner for our final-year medical students. Professor Linos studied in Athens and was then trained at the Harvard Medical School and the Mayo Clinic. As a world leading endocrine surgeon and a distinguished academic, Professor Linos has vast experience in guiding many young doctors in their careers. In this book, he provides "food for thought" to young people who are aspiring to become doctors. I have much pleasure in recommending this book and adding these short paragraphs on medicine in Hong Kong.

In 1887, Sir Patrick Manson founded the Hong Kong College of Medicine for Chinese, a forerunner to the School of Medicine of The University of Hong Kong.

Sir Patrick Manson was a Scottish physician renowned for his discoveries in tropical diseases. He was also a visionary with the desire to bring Western medicine to Hong Kong and Greater China. The Faculty of Medicine at The Chinese University of Hong Kong was inaugurated much later in 1982. Together, they represent the only two medical faculties in Hong Kong. Our medical schools are consistently ranked as being in the world's top 50, and admit only the top 1–2% of students based on their scores in public examinations.

At the turn of the century and under the British colonial rule, Hong Kong inherited a British or Commonwealth system of medical education. The city's undergraduate curriculum, residency and specialist training have for decades been very similar to those in the United Kingdom. To date, our specialist examinations continue to be all conjoined with the British and Australasian royal colleges. In anticipation of a change of sovereignty in 1997, the Hong Kong Academy of Medicine was formed with the objective to organize, monitor, assess and accredit specialist training and oversee the provision of continued medical education. Colleges with subspecialties subsequently formed.

People in Hong Kong have enjoyed excellent healthcare provided by our own medical graduates.

Our hospital system is similar to the National Health Service (NHS) of the United Kingdom and Canada. Public hospital services are provided at a minimal cost to our patients and with a high standard. Because Hong Kong is small in its size, patients can easily access hospitals. Our Chinese culture and values mean that the elderlies are looked after. Our government ensures good public health measures, including clean water and sanitation. All of the above contribute to the highest life expectancy among Hong Kong people in the world. The United Nations Vital Statistics Summary and Life Expectancy at Birth in 2016 reported an average of 87.3 years for women and 81.3 for men.

The path to becoming a physician is arduous. Medical students are required to assimilate a large wealth of knowledge, which is constantly evolving. At the same time, students learn to listen and be compassionate. Residency and specialist training take many years which demand diligence and dedication. Medical graduates here in Hong Kong, in addition, have the responsibility of maintaining the excellence of medical education under the "one country, two systems" arrangement. Healthcare in China is undergoing reforms, with an emphasis on primary care. With growing affluence, China is making significant strides in biomedical research. The number of publications from China in top-notch medical journals has been substantially increasing in recent years. Hong Kong medical graduates need to embrace what the two systems can offer, be international in their outlook, and be active in their academic pursuits.

At the inauguration ceremony of the Hong Kong College of Medicine for Chinese, Sir Manson suggested that Hong Kong should become "a center and a distributor, not for merchandise only, but also for science." He went on to suggest that we shall confer a boon on China and that medicine in Hong Kong should continue to contribute to its counterpart in Greater China.

I'm sure that you will find Professor Linos' book enjoyable. His writings will inspire those who want to become physicians and find echoes in the minds of those who have already taken on medicine as a career.

**Professor James Lau** is the Chairman of Department of Surgery, The Chinese University of Hong Kong.

# FOREWORD

Brian H. H. Lang

To those fortunate enough to have picked up this book and decided to read it, let me assure you that you are in for a treat. To me, this has to be one of the most honestly written guides in medicine with the simple intention of helping young, enthusiastic individuals wanting to pursue a medical career. This book will, however, appeal to a much wider audience, from high school students, medical students, internists, residents and qualified doctors, to even medical professors. Many of the valuable recommendations and advice made in these pages are extremely relevant and applicable across many different medical disciplines and subspecialties. To put it simply, this book is about helping each and every one of us to become a better medical student or a more effective physician. As one reads this book, there is a strong, inevitable feeling that this was written by an insider, someone who is clearly familiar with the "dos and don'ts" of how to be admitted into a top medical school, become successful, and become, as the author states in the book, "the best physician in the world."

However, this should not come as a surprise to anyone because this book was written by Professor Dimitrios Linos, a world-renowned and highly respected professor whose expertise is endocrine surgery. Apart from being a highly skilled and innovative surgeon, he was bestowed the presidency of the International Association of Endocrine Surgeons (IAES), which is one of the most prestigious societies in his surgical subspecialty. Therefore, there is little doubt that he has achieved what many surgeons could only aspire to achieve, and has remained at the pinnacle of his medical career. I am extremely grateful that he has decided to share his vast medical experience and astute observations in this wonderful book. I believe there is no one else who is as qualified as he is when it comes to giving such recommendations and advice to anyone aspiring to be a physician.

**Professor Brian Lang** is the Director of the Surgical Skills Training Center at the Department of Surgery, The University of Hong Kong.

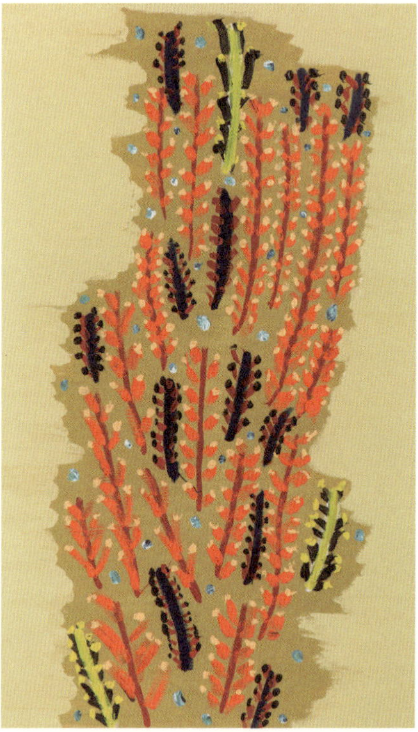

# INTRODUCTION

So you've decided to become a physician.
Are congratulations in order?
I'm not so sure.

Yes, you'll know the joy of curing pain; yes, you'll save lives; yes, your patients and their families will be grateful; and yes, there'll be times when you'll feel like a god.

No, you won't become rich; no, you won't be a very good parent; no, your sleepless nights at your patient's bedside will not be appreciated; no, you'll never really get to enjoy your holidays.

You may know the triumph of palm branches scattered at your feet as you enter Jerusalem, but you may also know betrayal at the hands of the very patients you benefited. And you may even experience your own crucifixion, with few chances of resurrection.

But at least, since you've decided to become a physician, make sure you're a good one!

The best physician in the world!

# BE THE BEST WOMAN PHYSICIAN IN THE WORLD

In most medical schools in the world today, the number of women is higher than the number of male medical students.

At Harvard Medical School, the leading medical school in the world and the most difficult to enter, in 2019, 165 students were accepted (out of 6,185 candidates), of whom 73 (44%) were men and 92 (56%) women.

But statistics show that for some "strange" reason, men eventually occupy the most important positions in medicine. A study in the prestigious journal *JAMA: The Journal of the American Medical Association*, showed that the academic staff in US medical schools consists of 30,464 women and 60,609 men. Full professors numbered 3,623 (11.9%) women and 17,354 (28.6%) men.

According to another major study published in *The BMJ*, the official journal of the British Medical Association, there were statistically more male department leaders in various medical specialties than women in the top 50 US medical schools funded by the National Institute of Health (NIH). Only seven medical schools and five specialties had more than 20% female leaders. Humorously titled "Plenty of Mustaches but Not Enough Women: Cross-sectional Study of Medical Leaders," this article reflects today's reality, which is slowly improving.

In particular, mothers who are physicians are more discriminated against than other working women, as described in another recent article in *The BMJ*. The study questioned 947 mothers who reported lower pay, fewer promotions to senior management, lack of support during pregnancy and the postpartum period, and difficulty in maintaining a balance between work and family responsibilities. Other studies report a different attitude towards a female physician by the patients themselves, whether they be male or female!

My own experience is that a young woman who decides to pursue medicine can become "the best physician in the world" while at the same time being the best partner and the best mother. My wife, Athena, whom I met when we were both medical students, has succeeded in all three areas, as have many other women who went to college with us. Of course it is true that until she was appointed full professor of epidemiology and Director of the Epidemiology Lab at Athens University's Medical School, she suffered relentless attacks, from which, however, she emerged ultimately triumphant. Her research work is internationally recognized and she is considered one of the most eminent Public Health Professors in Greece and abroad. Some of her published academic papers in America led to the enactment of laws banning pesticides that caused leukemia in farmers. Her other studies in Greece, in the industrial area of Oinofyta, north of Athens, caused countries and states such as California to ban "hexavalent chromium" in their drinking water. Besides her academic work, she has been recognized for her social and charity work, which every "best physician in the world" must carry out in parallel to his or her career. She has developed and run the Nutrition Program, which has been implemented throughout Greece for many years in order to feed and educate school children from vulnerable families. It has been recognized and awarded by institutions ranging from *The New York Times* to major Greek and international organizations.

Athena's effort to become the "best physician in the world" did not prevent her from becoming "the best mother in the world." She raised five children, all of whom were accepted at Harvard. Our four girls quickly became professors at Berkeley, Stanford and Harvard, demonstrating that if a woman decides to go down a difficult path, she can succeed.

The considerable difficulties faced by a young woman who wants to become a physician should not daunt her or hamper her deep desire to help her fellow humans through medicine. In fact, these difficulties will make it "easier" for her to finally become the "best physician in the world"!

# A WORD TO PARENTS

## Don't Pressure Your Child Into Becoming a Physician

As you read this book, you will realize that a physician's journey from beginning to end is tough and demanding, with many joyful moments but also many sorrows. Don't pressure your son or daughter into becoming a physician!

I've come across many types of "pressure," both direct and indirect, starting with "I'll make him into a physician" all the way to "we're not pushing him but . . ." Especially when one or both parents are physicians, their child's choice not to pursue medicine becomes increasingly diminished. These parents will eventually succeed in making their child into a physician, usually thanks to the various English-language profit-driven medical schools in Europe, but they will never understand such a physician's long-standing "disadvantage."

The inner knowledge that "I'm doing something I really don't like" and that I "got my degree because my parents begged and pressured me to get it," stays with them throughout their lives.

Of course there are those few who react before it's too late and who, after getting their medical degree and making their parents happy, go on to do what they truly love, becoming entrepreneurs, artists or politicians.

Most, however, continue on a passionless career in medicine, often choosing the same specialty as their physician parent. Even if the parent is a well-known and successful physician in his or her field, the struggle to match or exceed the parent's reputation creates additional psychological problems for the young physician. The pressure to become a physician can lead to a degree in medicine, to a medical specialty, and to continuing the family tradition, but it will never lead to self-esteem, which is one of the secrets of a truly successful physician.

## Stand By Your Child

On the other hand, if you feel that your child wants—and has what it takes—to go down the long and difficult road of becoming "the best physician in the world," then stand by him or her with all your might!

This means that your free time is now devoted to preparing your son or daughter in the best way possible to be admitted to a top medical school. You can no longer afford the luxury of going on vacation, enjoying your personal time or the good things in life. Instead, you devote yourself to finding the best tutor in higher mathematics, physics, and biology. You support your children throughout their school years in their athletic or artistic endeavors. You encourage them and help them highlight their leadership skills and charitable activities. You protect them from the "bad" school, and the "bad" professor. Know that your children "are always right." If your child tells you that a certain teacher is not helping them but instead is making things difficult for them, then they are right and you must protect them. If necessary, don't hesitate to take them to another school in the middle of the school year!

Do not be afraid of the financial problems that will arise until that incomparable day when you finally see your son or daughter graduate from medical school. There are so many scholarships and financial support mechanisms available, that even if you are financially less well off, you will succeed. As I advise below, some of the world's leading universities, such as Harvard, fully cover all costs (tuition, accommodation, food) for all eligible students whose parents earn less than $65,000 a year.

Support from both parents, offered discreetly—without interfering with your son or daughter's individual choices, without embarrassing them to their friends and acquaintances, and without telling them what to write in the personal statement that will accompany their application to university—is necessary while your child attends elementary, junior high and high school. Once they become med students, your "obligations" are diminished. Once they have "flown away" academically and professionally, then you will have all the time in the world to rest or to continue the same difficult but profoundly rewarding path of supporting your other children.

# A WORD TO TEACHERS

The school kids for whom I am writing this book are the pupils who will be admitted to medical schools such as Harvard, Cambridge or Oxford. He or she is not your ordinary student.

It might be the "nerd" who, ever since elementary school, has been the best student in the class, but it can also be the "misbehaving one," the "indifferent one," or the "bad" student who causes problems in the classroom. I would like to talk to you about this student, who may in fact be a "gifted child" and who needs to be quickly discovered and supported.

These children, the so-called "charismatic" ones, from a very young age use a rich vocabulary, ask persistent questions, and engage in discussions with adults. They have an amazing memory and can repeat something word for word, days after hearing it. They can solve problems very quickly, with a different way of thinking than usual. When they are interested in a topic, they focus and study it in depth. On the contrary, when an issue does not challenge or interest them, they grow bored and show it, often disappearing into their room or into places where they can enjoy their isolation.

At school, because they are not intellectually stimulated by the standard educational process, they can become "problematic" children. Some researchers have observed that charismatic boys in particular have no fondness for their school or their teachers. Unlike charismatic girls who are usually considered star pupils, charismatic boys tend not to do their homework for the next day and are generally regarded as misfits.

A good and experienced teacher should identify these children, offer them more challenges, and make them their "partners" in teaching the other students. The hoped-for outcome is to win them over by recognizing their particular mental abilities, but of course without discriminating against the other pupils in the class.

Behind every successful physician is a teacher who believed in them and supported them, especially when the other teachers were indifferent or even obstructed the child's schooling.

A good physician, "the best physician in the world," is yet another gift from a good educator to his or her country.

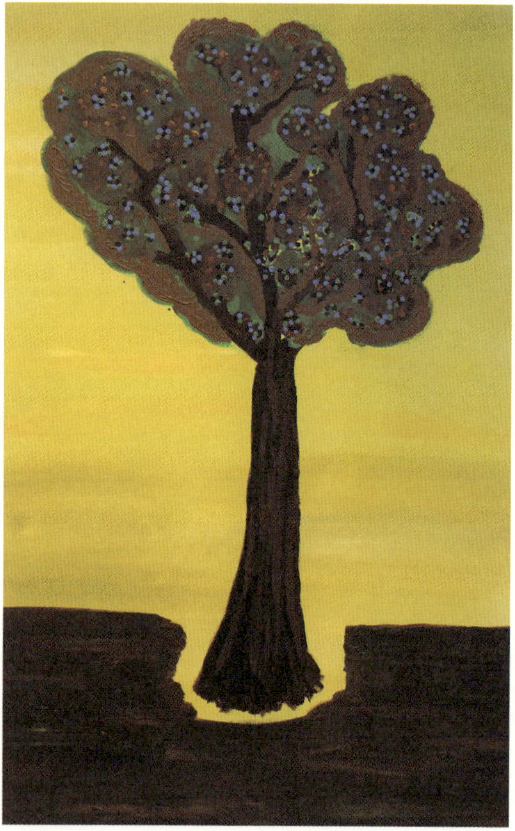

# A GOOD MEDICAL SCHOOL

Choosing a good medical school is the first step to becoming a good physician, and indeed one of the best physicians in the world.

The medical schools in your country are your first choice. You could get into one of those and then go on to specialize at one of the most renowned universities in the world. That is how the majority of today's most prominent physicians abroad started out. They completed basic medical studies in their home country and then managed to continue at one or more internationally recognized centers elsewhere. George Papanikolaou graduated from the Athens Medical School before ending up at Cornell University in New York and working there on the technique that was later named after him, the Papanicolaou or Pap test, which has saved millions of women from cervical cancer.

If you are a very good student in junior high and high school, or even if you are not a straight-A student but are a charismatic kid who knows a lot, learns much faster than the other kids in class, and is bored and frustrated at school, it is worth thinking about applying to the internationally recognized top medical schools.

We all know which the best medical schools in the world are, and we also know how very difficult it is to be accepted by them. In Europe, besides Cambridge and Oxford medical schools, other medical schools in England are considered very good, which is why international competition for admission is intense. Applying to these schools in England requires special preparation, which should start early.

Unlike in Europe, where a candidate for medical school is a high school graduate, in the United States a candidate for medical school is a graduate of a four-year college.

While in Europe you can get your degree in medicine after six years of studies, in the United States the minimum time is eight years. In addition to the very stringent process of admission to college, one must undergo an even more demanding process in order to be admitted to medical school, part of which is the MCAT (Medical College Admission Test).

So then a logical question would be: "Why not finish med school in Europe in six years and then pursue a specialty in the United States, instead of trying to finish med school in the United States after at least eight years?"

The answer, as we shall see later, is that the best American centers and universities that offer medical specialty training prefer US medical school graduates. Thus, the most formidable graduates of Europe's internationally renowned medical schools are obliged to undergo additional training or to carry out additional research at a US university before being able to specialize. Therefore, what started off as six years turn into at least eight before graduates or students can move on to where both their potential and their heart drive them.

The great benefit of entering med school later in the United States compared to Europe is that it enables the prospective physician to make this decision at a more mature age.

If the thought of being a physician for the rest of your life doesn't really excite you, if the pressure of your parents—especially those who are physicians themselves—is overwhelming, then the delayed choice of a graduate school of medicine in America will help you make your final decision. Conversely, if the desire to serve your fellow humans through medicine grew while you were studying another science, now is your chance to pursue a four-year graduate degree in medicine. Besides those in the United States, similar graduate medical schools exist in other countries and continents.

If in the end you don't get admitted into any of your country's medical schools, if you are unable to get into the difficult English medical schools, and if you're not considering the US process, then the question of whether you should study at one of the numerous for-profit English-speaking medical schools in Cyprus, Romania, the Czech Republic, Hungary, etc., becomes imperative. My advice would be to carefully examine the school's international rankings in order to choose the most internationally recognized ones that demonstrably allow their graduates to pursue their specialization at the best universities in the United States and Europe. The advertising—and often misleading—

messages of these for-profit English-speaking medical schools may get you enrolled in medical school very easily. But the road from then on will be a difficult one. Your specialty training is directly related to the medical school you graduated from. The best universities and internationally acclaimed hospitals and centers for medical specialization select candidates from the best medical schools and, as we will see later, there is tough competition among many candidates from many medical schools around the world for just a few positions to train in medical specialties.

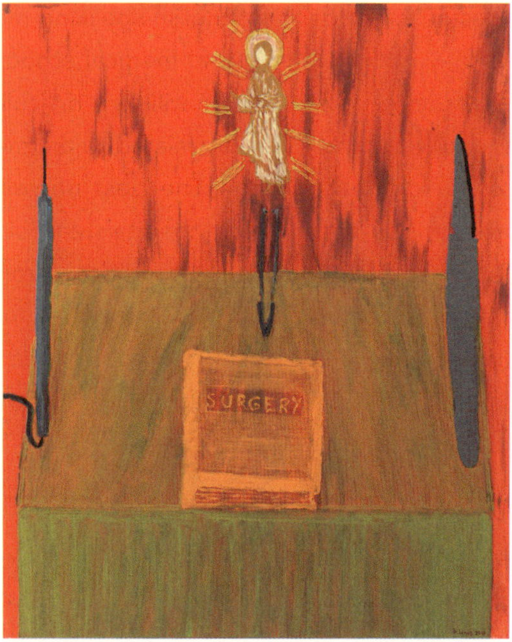
SURGERY

# PREPARING FOR MEDICAL SCHOOLS IN THE USA

If you are a straight-A student, a good athlete, a promising painter, or a leader in a school community that carries out innovative philanthropic activities, then it is well worth your time to prepare for one of the best universities in the world, which will in turn open the door to one of the world's best medical schools: Harvard Medical School. Of course, the same preparation may lead you to Stanford, Yale or Johns Hopkins and one of their world-famous medical schools.

There is no recipe for getting into Harvard. The Director of Admissions who decides who will finally be admitted says: "We hope to attract and accept students of every imaginable background and every kind of preparation."

The things I will briefly mention below are based on my own experience of preparing our five children, who were all admitted to Harvard. I hasten to add that the only one who became a physician was Eleni, who is now Professor of Dermatology at Stanford.

## Your Grades

The role grades play in being admitted to Harvard can be seen indirectly on the university's website, which explains the selection process and the criteria observed by the commission that studies each candidate's application: "We want to accept students with dynamism, talent and diversity who will be able to make a significant contribution to the education of their peers." Furthermore, "the majority of students admitted represent a range of scores from roughly 600 to 800 on each section of the SAT as well as on the SAT Subject Tests." Our daughter Elizabeth took the SAT for the first time when she was 12 years old. Her results at the time were Verbal 650 and Math 720, but later on, she improved her Verbal score to 720. Her SAT Subject Tests results were Literature 710, Math IIC 760, Physics 780, and Writing 800.

In addition to the SAT exams, a candidate can also take the AP (Advanced Placement) exams, with the highest score being 5. At Harvard and at other major US universities, if a candidate has a 5 in four difficult courses, then she or he is allowed to graduate in three instead of four years. This is especially important for those who are considering going on to medical schools. In the USA, with good grades in your AP exams, you can finish your medical studies in seven years. Our first daughter, Katerina, had an AP score of 5 in six subjects (Biology, English Lit and Composition, Chemistry, French, Calculus AB, and US History), yet she chose to attend all four years of Harvard University and not pursue a medical degree.

In Greece and many other European countries, besides the SAT, the SAT II, and the AP exams, there are also the IB (International Baccalaureate) exams, the results of which are also recognized in the United States as objective examinations for the evaluation of a candidate. The early acquisition of High Level IB certificates prior to submitting applications to US universities instead of teachers' predictions is another "secret weapon" that will reinforce a candidate's application in terms of grades.

## Your Personal Statement

If good grades are a prerequisite, the personal statement is the next most important factor in whether or not a student is admitted to Harvard or any other top US university. This essay helps the admissions committee get to know you in ways unrelated to courses, grades, exam results, and other objective criteria. It will show your ability to organize your thoughts and express yourself. "We're looking for an essay that will help us get to know you better as a person and a student," according to Harvard University's website. In her personal statement, my daughter Katerina wrote about the "right to be undecided," a right that should be granted to every student who is considering medicine as a lifelong career. A personal statement must be precisely "personal," with perhaps just the slightest advisory intervention by a parent on the final draft. Members of the admissions committee can easily tell when a personal statement has actually been written by the candidate and when it is the result of someone else's work.

## Letters of Recommendation

Letters of recommendation are an important part of the acceptance or rejection process of a candidate's application to Harvard. As it states on their website, "they can illuminate such personal qualities as character and leadership, as well as intellectual curiosity, creativity, and love of learning."

Here too, much care is needed. Candidates should ask for a letter of recommendation from someone who knows them well, someone for whom they have been working for quite some time. One of the most powerful letters of recommendation for one of our daughters was written by a woman in charge of an orphanage. The letter described how important it was to the children that our daughter went there for an hour every week and taught them to sing English songs. Letters of recommendation from prime ministers, archbishops and other important public figures whom the parents may know have the exact opposite result: The admissions committee can see straight away that the praise is intended for the parent and not their son or daughter, and the application is rejected.

In 2019, Harvard received 43,330 applications. Of those, 1,950 were accepted, i.e., 4.5%. Of those, about 10% were from other countries. Every year, for example, an average of just one or two students from Greece are accepted into Harvard College. The percentage of US college graduates admitted to Harvard Medical School in 2019 was 3.3%. In any case, percentages refer to the many. But you are unique; you are the one who has decided to become "the best physician in the world." Aim for the top and you will surely achieve great heights, and this journey will be worth it from its first to its very last day. In this book you will read about some of the difficulties you will encounter and my suggestions for overcoming them.

One of the major difficulties for undergraduate and postgraduate studies in the USA is the high cost, especially when compared to the corresponding costs in other countries, or to Europe in general. The good news, though, is that if you finally succeed and are admitted to Harvard or another top US university, all your expenses—annual tuition, room and board—could be fully covered by the university. At Harvard, if your parents' annual income is less than $65,000 a year, you pay nothing. If their income is slightly higher, you will pay a correspondingly smaller percentage of the costs borne by the children of wealthy families.

Similarly, when you graduate from college and are admitted to one of the top US medical schools, there are ways of tackling the financial problem for four years of study. Recently, the NYU School of Medicine decided that all medical students should study tuition-free. At Harvard Medical School, more than $37 million is distributed annually to over 72% of students in the form of scholarships, job opportunities, and loans. The government grants loans of up to $40,000 a year to each student. In recent years, efforts have been made to reduce the financial cost of education in the USA. Even so, I believe that the long-term benefits of a good education at the best American universities can partially justify the high costs borne by those students who ultimately do not enjoy the financial relief mentioned above.

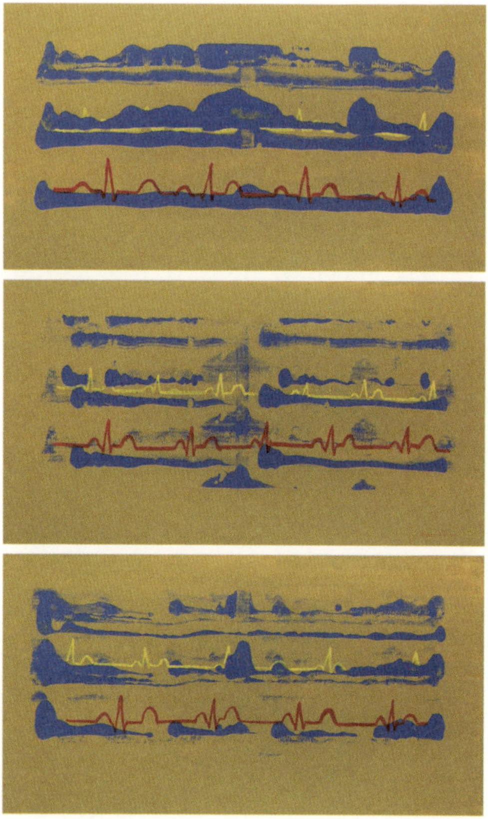

# PREPARING FOR MEDICAL SCHOOLS IN THE UK

There are more than 30 medical schools in the United Kingdom (UK). Some of them, such as the ones at Cambridge and Oxford, rank among the top 10 medical schools in the world.

Graduates of these medical schools are more readily accepted to pursue a medical specialty at one of America's internationally recognized hospitals and institutes, which is why the competition for admission to one of the UK's medical schools is fierce. The preparation of a good student who is thinking of studying medicine in the UK must start early on and be very methodical.

## Your Grades

As in all medical schools, grades in the last years of high school as well as the separate, objective entrance exams are the basic requirement for a candidate's admission to medical school.

Applicants to British medical schools must have high grades in their GCSE (General Certificate of Secondary Education) courses, which are taken by students aged 14–16 years. In fact, they need A+ and A grades in at least five science courses (Chemistry, Physics, Biology), Mathematics and English to get into most good medical schools.

Similarly, high grades in the IB Baccalaureate system can lead to medical schools. Here too, candidates with three or more A levels in Biology, Physics, Chemistry, Mathematics or similar subjects at the higher level and with a grade of 7 in the IB system are likely to be accepted to top British medical schools.

In addition to good school grades, three admissions tests are offered to candidates by most medical schools. The UCAT (University Clinical Aptitude Test) exams are required at 25 medical schools, including King's College London, Edinburgh University and Glasgow University. The UCAT exams focus on questions of varying difficulty that must be answered in a short amount of time. They cover topics from verbal reasoning, quantitative reasoning and abstract reasoning, to situational judging and the like.

The BMAT (BioMedical Admissions Test) is required by seven medical schools including Cambridge, Oxford, and Imperial College. In the BMAT, the emphasis is on mathematics, the sciences, and reasoning.

Finally, the GAMSAT (Graduate Medical School Admission Test) is designed for holders of a recognized Bachelor's degree who wish to study medicine at British universities offering four-year graduate entry programs.

## Personal Statement

As with applications for admission to the top US universities, in the UK as well, a candidate's personal statement plays a major role in the committee's decision to accept—to make an offer to—a prospective medical student. In fact, if your school and tests grades aren't the best, an outstanding personal statement can help significantly.

The members of a university's admissions committee, who read hundreds of applications and personal statements from prospective students from the UK and other countries around the world, have to be impressed by your desire to help your suffering fellow human beings and to study contemporary medical dilemmas more profoundly. They have to be able to see that you are passionate about becoming a physician.

Generalizations such as "helping the patient" or "being involved in the progress of science" do not help unless they are accompanied by specific actions and activities to date. Specific obstacles in your personal life that you have been able to overcome, and collaborations and initiatives that show that you can be both a leader and a team player, will give an edge to your personal statement and lend support to your application to medical school. Exaggerations, generalizations, and essays that are not truly personal can lead to your application being rejected, especially if your grades are not stellar. "Personal" also means that you wrote the statement yourself and that it was not written by a parent or your British university applications advisor. Of course, sharing your statement with these people and asking for their input is useful, and you should do it.

## The Interview

When you are invited for an interview, you know that you are already close to the realization of your dream of being admitted to a British medical school.

From the point of view of the admissions committee, which will decide who to eventually accept, it is a unique opportunity to not only confirm what you have written in your application and your personal statement, but also to evaluate your communication skills, a necessary quality in a future physician. At most medical schools, interviews aim to discover who you really are, why you want to become a physician, and what your ambitions are.

In certain medical schools such as Cambridge and Oxford, the discussion will be more "scientific." They will want to assess your broader knowledge and your ability to synthesize and provide scientifically sound solutions, even if you don't know the correct answer to the question asked. In other words, don't say "I don't know"—instead continue to answer based on the parts of the question you do know and make reasonable inferences that are likely to benefit humanity. For instance, if they ask you "how do butterflies mate?", you shouldn't become flustered but rather start with facts about fertilization that you are familiar with from biology and continue with sensible suggestions to which those who asked the question could have no scientific objections. I still remember my surprise at being told about a similar question on "bee mating" my daughter Eleni was asked in her Cambridge interview before being accepted to Trinity College. I also remember how long her interview lasted compared to other candidates who, within ten minutes, would leave the room, obviously disappointed at their performance. Keeping your cool and being confident that you are well prepared will help your interview be an enjoyable experience on your way to a British medical school.

# YOU ARE NOW A MEDICAL STUDENT

Whichever six-year medical school you have been admitted to, either in your home country or elsewhere in Europe, there are two things you should bear in mind:

1. Continue to be one of the best students in medical school as you were, for many years, in your previous studies, and
2. Make sure you take the first step to take the United States Medical Licensing Examination (USMLE) no later than your fourth year of medical school.

Diligently attending and studying for all your courses, preparing for and taking exams in a timely manner, studying the most internationally acclaimed textbooks (and not whatever textbooks your professors may have written) will help you prepare for the USMLE at the same time.

I suggest that you take the USMLE exams early, even if you have not yet decided whether you will go on to study in the United States. It is an objective assessment that certifies your ability in any country to which you decide to apply for your residency.

Many first-year students, tired after their effort to succeed in the previous year's entrance exams, relax too much and end up accumulating academic obligations that are difficult to fulfil later. You need to take care and use your common sense to keep from getting physically exhausted and to not fall too far behind in the beginning.

Of course, student life offers different opportunities, not only for one's academic but also for one's intellectual development. It is a unique opportunity for you as a student to discover fine music, painting and sculpture, good literature and poetry. You may have the chance to visit some of the most unique places in the world (such as Po Lin Monastery in Lantau Island in

Hong Kong, or St. Anthony's Monastery in the Sonoran Desert of Arizona in the US) and get to know some remarkable people who will help you answer the most profound and difficult questions about your life.

Your new friends at medical school and your teachers at all levels will always have something new to teach you. Get to know them better. Most medical students are soon fascinated by the clinical specialties of surgery, cardiology, pediatrics, and psychiatry. Fewer get excited about microbiology, anatomic pathology or the other "laboratory" specialties.

But you now have the opportunity as a student to discover the joys and potential of another kind of medicine, one that focuses not on the individual but on the many. Public health, epidemiology, social medicine, and global health, as we shall see later, are new challenges for an accomplished medical student.

Prepare yourself in time for the next step in your journey to become the best physician in the world. As I said before, your success in the USMLE before you get your medical degree makes it much easier for you to take the next right step, that is, to be accepted into the best training program for the specialty you have chosen, not only in the United States but anywhere in the world. Take advantage of the medical students exchange programs. Visit other medical schools in other countries around the world.

If you are not from the US, the chance to spend a couple of months with US medical students and get to know the high level of US clinical and laboratory medicine early on is invaluable. You'll discover new areas of medicine in which you could later specialize. You'll be introduced to the—by and large internationally acclaimed—professors at the hospital where you could be working as a foreign visiting medical student. If you impress them at this time with your hard work, your ethics, your knowledge and especially your daily smile, you'll build up a strong lead as a future applicant for training at the hospital's residency program, which is your next objective.

# YOU ARE NOW A MEDICAL DOCTOR: YOUR NEXT STEPS

The medical degree alone is not enough to become the best physician in the world. Specialization is your next step.

I'm sure that in any country there are very good centers for training in all medical specialties. I also know the top training centers in Europe, Asia, and Australia.

But today we all agree that residency programs in the United Sates are the ones that provide a young intern with the best education in a specific amount of training time, which is known in advance.

The dream of all new physicians and even professors of medicine around the world is to train fully or at least partially at one of America's renowned university hospitals.

The main reason for the superiority of the US residency programs is that from the first year they immediately "throw you in at the deep end," quickly making you into a self-reliant physician.

Let's take the specialty of surgery as an example. During the first year, the program is required to train you in order to allow you to perform simple surgeries on your own. Gradually in the second year, the operations become more complex, and so on. In fact, in your fifth year as Chief Resident you will have an independent team and the right to operate on your own.

It's one thing to do an appendectomy under the responsibility and supervision of someone else; it's quite another to have to come into direct contact with the anxious parents and their child who is suffering from abdominal pain, to decide that surgery is required, and to carry out that surgery yourself.

In Europe and elsewhere in the world, by contrast, the system for training young surgeons is different.

An intern, but also one who has completed his or her specialty and is considered a surgeon, has for many years been dependent on the guidance of a senior director or professor.

I'll never forget when, as a young assistant professor, I visited one of the top German university hospitals, which had a very famous German professor as its director of surgery. At 7:00 a.m., everyone would gather in the amphitheater and wait for the professor to announce the surgery schedule of the day. The professor would then supervise all the operating rooms, criticizing even older surgeons. I was impressed by everybody's total dependence on and adherence to the professor's choices. The hierarchy, as it applies in Europe, clearly is an impediment to new surgeons becoming quickly independent.

As a young resident graduating from an accredited US residency program, your self-confidence and your belief that you will indeed become the best physician in the world will be more than worth your efforts to be accepted into such a program.

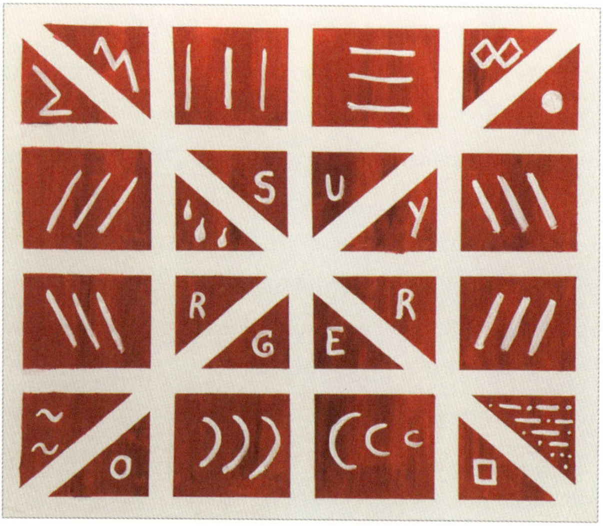
S U Y
R G E R

# PREREQUISITES FOR SPECIALIZING IN THE USA

The first prerequisite when starting your search for a US residency program is to have passed all three steps of the USMLE, as mentioned above.

If you haven't already passed Step 1 of the USMLE as a medical student, you need to immediately start studying for this first step of the examination, which is the most difficult, as it assesses knowledge you acquired in the first years of medical school. Steps 2 and 3 are easier. Once you pass the USMLE, which demonstrates that you have basic medical knowledge in accordance with US standards, you are eligible to participate in the process of selecting a training program in your chosen specialty.

The matching program, as the selection procedure is called, allows any medical specialty training program to select the candidates it wants, based on the list of candidates who have included it in their application.

Thanks to this system, renowned teaching hospitals, such as Massachusetts General, Stanford Health Care, the Mayo Clinic, the Cleveland Clinic and Johns Hopkins, select the best candidate physicians from around the world to join their residency programs. Because US medical school graduates are typically the best candidates due to their 8–10 years of studies to obtain a medical degree, they are the ones who will fill the positions in the most popular American residency programs in the various specialties.

But even if you graduated from a non-US medical school and are what they call an International Medical Graduate (IMG), don't let that stop you.

If you got high scores in the USMLE, if they met you as a medical student in a clinical clerkship (1–2 month training programs as a student at a US hospital), and if you have the right mentor who is known and respected in the USA, why not apply straight away to several hospitals through the matching program?

If you "dare" to embark on this process, be sure to apply for the "worst" programs, the ones that good American students would never apply to for residency. You may have been the best medical student in your country, and you might admire Harvard, Stanford, Yale and all the other internationally-recognized US universities, but the chances are very slim that you will be admitted there right after graduating from your homeland's medical school.

If you are accepted at one of the residency programs not preferred by the top graduates of US medical schools, then you can immediately start your US education in the specialty you have chosen and, of course, you can complete your compulsory study time earlier so that you can take your specialty exams, the famous "Boards," sooner. Only if you pass your Boards are you entitled to say that you were fully trained in your specialty in the United States. Your prospective patients and employers will duly appreciate this fact.

If you are a top graduate from a foreign medical school, believe me, the "worst" US training program might be better than the best one in your country. The reason for this is the strict central supervision of all certified US programs, so that everything is in the best interest of the intern. If, for instance, the new surgical intern is deprived of the chance to carry out an operation as a "first" surgeon by his professor or another senior surgeon who is in a hurry or considers the surgery "his" or "hers," then that hospital, however prestigious, is at risk of losing its license for training new surgeons. And that would be a serious blow to both its pride and its finances, which depend on government subsidies for the training of young surgeons.

As you finish this "second-best" residency program and, having proven that you are an extraordinary resident, you have high hopes of continuing and completing your residency or post-residency fellowship in a sub-specialty at one of the famous teaching hospitals and training programs that you always dreamed of (Harvard, Stanford, Johns Hopkins, etc.).

Alternatively (and this is what most IMGs do), before starting your specialty training program, you dedicate two to four years to medical research. In this way, through your publications, your presence at US medical conferences, and your personal acquaintance with leading figures in academic medicine, you will prove that, despite being an IMG, you deserve to pursue your specialty at one of the most renowned US academic programs. Research programs at distinguished teaching hospitals are also limited. Here is where your background as a student, your work in your home country with a physician who is known in America, and your personal presence at the interviews will all come in helpful.

If you choose this option, you are more likely to be admitted to a more acclaimed residency program, but at the same time you will obviously put back the day you will be able to take your Boards—the day you will finally become a specialist physician.

Another tip I would like to give you, if you are a graduate of a foreign university (but also if you are a graduate of a US medical school), is to try to enroll in a Master's of Public Health (MPH) program at one of the best public health schools in the United States. After one or two years of intensive study of fields such as epidemiology, biostatistics, or health economics, you will possess objective proof that you can contribute to the academic progress of the program that may accept you as an intern.

The director of any of the sought-after residency programs would look very favorably upon a candidate with a Harvard University Master's of Public Health degree, even if this candidate were an IMG.

Furthermore, attending a good public health school in America may open up a new opportunity you had never considered before. There are very few medical graduates pursuing a professional and academic career in public health. Most public health teachers are not physicians, and yet they make medical and health decisions for millions of citizens around the world.

Could it be that, with your training in medicine, you could become a public health professional, fighting the diseases that plague humanity today?

Are your initial thoughts of becoming a surgeon, a cardiologist, a gynecologist, or an ophthalmologist worth changing in order to offer more health to more of your fellow human beings around the world?

You decide!

# YOU ARE NOW A RESIDENT

The fact that you were admitted and can now begin your residency in the United States or in a good training center in Asia or Europe does not necessarily mean that you will be able to continue into the next year or even graduate and be eligible to take the exams for your chosen specialty. Indeed, in many well-known training programs in the United States, the "pyramid system" applies. The first year of residency in surgery begins with ten prospective surgeons, but in the end there are places for only four chief residents. During the second, third, and fourth year, the weakest residents will be forced to leave either the hospital or surgery.

Your behavior towards your patients, your colleagues, and the hospital staff, as well as your in-training examinations, will all contribute to the hospital's decision to allow you to continue your education in your chosen specialty.

There's only one secret to surviving and succeeding in your training in the specialty of your choice by completing the program, and that's: hard work!

My advice is, especially if you are a foreign graduate (IMG), to try to work harder than all your colleagues, and to do it with a smile, with patience, and with your vision always helping you stay strong and prudent.

No matter how many countries try to legislatively limit interns' formal training and hospital hours, a good physician is shaped by many hours in the operating room and at the hospital among the patients and the nursing staff.

When I was a surgical resident at the Mayo Clinic, I was on call every other night. This meant that I went home every other day for very few hours during the night. Even then, however, my limited sleep was interrupted by phone calls from the nurses asking for my approval to, for example, give a patient painkillers. I remember how rude and abrupt I was when answering those nighttime phone calls and how apologetic—and always bearing donuts—I was with the nurses the next morning.

Although such training programs are now illegal, there is no doubt that the more clinical activities you participate in as a resident, the greater your chances of becoming a good physician. The more you read the related literature and participate in clinical research during your basic education, the better a physician you'll become.

## Respect the Nursing Staff

One piece of advice that you should follow, from the very first day you start your residency program to the last day before you stop working, is to respect the nursing staff.

I still remember, as a first-year resident at the Mayo Clinic on duty in the Intensive Care Unit (ICU), the invaluable help of the nurses in administering medication to patients. I always listened to their opinion and judgment with respect, appreciation and humility.

In contrast, a colleague of mine, a first-year intern but a graduate of Harvard Medical School, could not understand how it was possible for a nurse to know more about something than he did. I assure you that while I spent those difficult weeks of my training in the ICU calmly and without any trouble, the same can't be said for him.

You should never argue with people just because that's what your ego dictates. Your good relations with the nursing staff, combined with your hard personal work, will allow you to continue and successfully complete your training program in the specialty you have chosen.

## Always Tell the Truth

Another very important piece of advice that you need to remember, both as an intern and as a young physician, but also as a mature physician, is to always tell the truth. Never try to not tell the whole truth or to embellish reality.

During your training, your senior physicians and professors will easily spot your omissions, your laziness, your mistakes. It's so much better for you to come clean and say "sorry, I didn't think of it," "I couldn't be bothered," or "I made a mistake," than to try to hide all or part of the truth.

The detailed recording and admission of your wrong choices or omissions, no matter how painful it may be at first, is the only real solution to any of your problems during your medical career, and the only thing that will give you relief. Please never forget that.

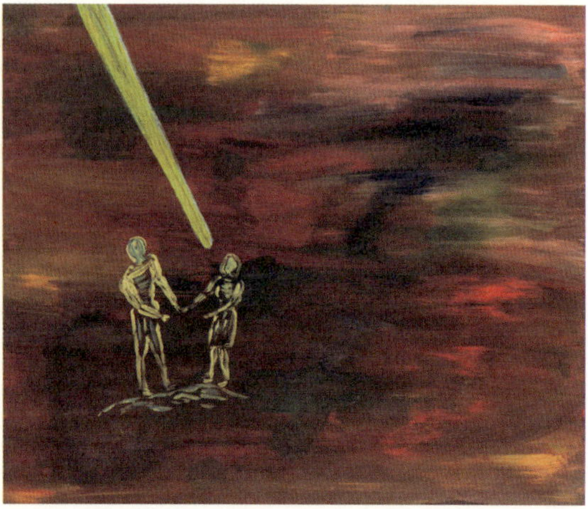

# THE PHYSICIAN-PATIENT RELATIONSHIP

From the first days of your residency, you will have savored the unique experience of the doctor's relationship with the patient. It is a relationship that will set an indelible seal on your life. It is a relationship that cannot be described in words. Just as there are no words to describe love, there are no words to describe the sacred relationship between physician and patient. It is a relationship that will become the center of your life, a relationship that will give you the greatest joys—and inevitably the greatest sorrows—in your life.

It is truly a deeply committed relationship, which, however, has its own rules.

Hippocrates set the first of these rules in his famous oath, in the $4^{th}$ century B.C. "I will not give a lethal drug to anyone if I am asked, nor will I advise such a plan; and similarly I will not give a woman a pessary to cause an abortion. Into whatever homes I go, I will enter them for the benefit of the sick, avoiding any voluntary act of impropriety or corruption, including the seduction of women or men, whether they are free men or slaves. Whatever I see or hear in the lives of my patients, whether in connection with my professional practice or not, which ought not to be spoken of outside, I will keep secret, as considering all such things to be private. In purity and according to divine law will I carry out my life in my art."

Today, the rules of the relationship between physician and patient have become more and more complex. Today most doctors don't practice solo medicine. They can't give their patients the time that they and their patients would like. Today most doctors are obliged to become members of managed care organizations. These organizations require the doctor to be more "productive" by seeing as many patients as possible in the shortest amount of time. Patients feel they are on a conveyor belt with a production-line oriented physician. Hospital administrations, insurance companies, and new state regulations require doctors to deal more with bureaucracy than with their patients.

On the other hand, before visiting their doctor, most patients have visited the Internet. The absolute confidence patients used to have in their doctors is a thing of the past. The classic paternalistic approach in which the doctor decided what was best for the patient only applies in emergency situations, when there isn't the time to obtain consent from the patient.

The informative or interpretive model are alternative approaches that require the physician to act as a technical expert or advisor, with the patient making the final decision regarding the treatment of his or her medical condition.

I prefer the so-called "fourth model of physician-patient relationship," the deliberative approach. The physician remains a friend and teacher, explaining the optimal medical measures for each case. The patient's consent remains important for the implementation of treatment.

When I am asked my medical opinion by Maria, Helen, Andrew or Peter, I have already become Maria, Helen, Andrew or Peter before answering. I ask myself, "If I were the patient, how would I like the doctor to talk to me?" And this gives me the strength and the way to talk to each person according to their ability to fully understand the scientific steps and decisions that I would take if I were that person.

Establishing such a relationship with your patient, i.e., putting their interests first, will protect you and is a safe guide. Even if later on you find yourself in the difficult position of having to explain a medical error or a complication, the same honest and transparent relationship should be maintained. Don't ever hesitate at such a crucial moment—which you are bound to face in your medical career—to give early reporting and analysis of the mishap, full explanations to the patient and family, and emotional support, apologies and compensation if at fault.

Studies suggest that transparent accountability is better for everyone involved in the long run. Most patients will appreciate such an approach by their physician.

The physician-patient relationship should be kept alive in both good and bad times. This is your oxygen. Without an honest and loving relationship with your patients, you cannot continue to be "the best physician in the world!"

# YOU ARE NOW A BOARD CERTIFIED PHYSICIAN

So you've completed your residency in your chosen specialty. You're about to become a Board Certified physician.

You are ready to choose the type of medicine you wish to practice. These are your options:

## Academic Medicine

If are reading this book, chances are you've already decided to pursue a career in academic medicine.

Most likely you were a grade A student in high school and belonged to the group of top medical students. Indeed, if you were lucky enough to come across an exemplary academic professor, you probably caught the bug and aspire to one day become like that professor or even better.

During your residency, the desire to pursue academic medicine will either remain and perhaps grow more ardent, or other more "sensible" thoughts will lead you to other options.

Academic medicine will give you the unique opportunity—the joy, to be precise—of being among students and young physicians, waiting like open-mouthed, fledgling sparrows to receive their intellectual sustenance from you.

The experience of talking to many students at once but also one-on-one can inspire great devotion and commitment. You offer all you can to the student you have in front of you, without expecting anything in return. Your greatest delight is to see these students get ahead in medicine and do well in their courses and exams. In fact, if some of them want to work with you in their spare time and eventually go on to add their name to yours as co-authors of a published paper, this relationship becomes even stronger.

The students, be they few or many, who have honored you with their respect and trust, will become your spiritual children and will give you joy for many years to come, even when you are old and have retired from active medicine.

Academic medicine also offers you the unique satisfaction of contributing to the progress of medicine through your research, published articles and papers at international conferences.

The international recognition of your clinical and research work is an unprecedented experience. Seeing a paper of yours published in a leading scientific journal is an incomparable thrill that is impossible to describe. At that moment you forget all the sleepless nights, the hard work, the sacrifices you made for months to gather the research material, to analyze it, to then write the paper, to send it to the medical journal of your choice, to have it rejected, to rewrite it and then resubmit it for publication. For an academic physician, an academic paper acceptance letter means more than anyone outside academic medicine can imagine, and it will leave your "sensible" friend wondering if it was worth all that effort.

When their colleagues and friends are relaxing on weekends, academic physicians are working on their next paper. When they receive messages from friends holidaying in Phuket, they are busy travelling to Bangkok to attend international conferences. Deep down they know the bitter truth that it makes absolutely no difference whether the hotel hosting the conference they are attending from 7:30 in the morning until 7:30 at night is located in Greece, the Caribbean, China, or Australia. On the other hand, their academic life gives them more joy than any vacation might.

Academic life has its joys but it is also fiercely competitive, often unethically so. Envy of your academic success can lead your rivals to extreme actions. "Your death, my life" is an experience you will not be spared.

Now here are some tips to help you avoid the negative aspects of academic medicine.

First of all, keep a low profile in everything you do. You don't have to talk about yourself and your successes. Let others speak for you. Be careful not to get carried away by bad and unethical academic habits. The data and analysis of your findings should always be true. Don't steal someone else's idea, for instance one that you read about as a reviewer for a journal.

Don't collaborate with academic physicians if you question the truthfulness and validity of their findings. It's better to produce a smaller number of papers that truly reflect your personal work and research.

Never forget that, sooner or later, "truth will out." You would not wish to be stigmatized academically, because even if it does not cost you your academic advancement, at the end of the day your personal pain will be greater than the joy of your false success. We can fool all of the people some of the time, but not ourselves.

## Public Hospital

As a public hospital physician, you'll have hardly any academic obligations (such as student education, research and writing), but perhaps more clinical work.

Public hospitals serve many patients, especially those with limited financial means. In most countries, public hospitals are worse off in terms of facilities and working conditions than private or purely university hospitals.

The difficulties may be greater, but the joys of a physician working in a public hospital and helping his or her fellow humans, who are invariably poor and unknown, may be greater than those of an academic or private physician.

Even though you are not required to produce academic work at the same time that you are working as a clinician, you could inspire and organize academic opportunities in the public hospital, for example by initiating collaboration with the nearest university and starting to educate medical students. Your participation in national and international research protocols and your presence at international medical conferences will improve your life.

By working in a public hospital, you will have the chance to become one of the best physicians in the world.

## Private Hospital

Places for physicians in university or public hospitals may be limited, so that the new physician may have no other choice but to go into private medicine. Medicine in a private hospital offers many opportunities and prospects. First of all, there is the feeling of freedom to do what you want when you want and how you want—to be able to be your own boss.

Of course, this is an illusion, because in private medicine there are difficulties just as there are in academic and public medicine. Instead of the dean, here you have to deal with the director of the private hospital. Instead of your limited academic or state salary, here there are the restrictions of private insurance companies that decide how much you will be paid for a medical procedure, regardless of the quality of your education or experience. Rivalries among your colleagues in private medicine are no less bitter than the ones you encounter in academic or public medicine.

But it is true that in private medicine you may have more time for yourself and your family, which is a very important factor for your mental equilibrium and happiness. This important possibility alone is worth the decision of the specialist to pursue private medicine.

Practicing private medicine does not prevent you from savoring some of the joys of academic medicine. Medical students from the local university or other medical schools in your country or abroad can be trained by you if you so desire and can prove that you mean to dedicate time to your visiting students.

Clinical studies—and indeed, ones that can have an international impact—can easily be carried out at a private hospital. As an example, I will mention the studies of the internationally renowned surgeon Akira Miyauchi on the possibility that small papillary thyroid cancer can be treated without surgery, only through active surveillance. These clinical studies, which are the only ones of their kind in the international literature of the field and have influenced international guidelines, were performed at the privately-owned Kuma Hospital in Japan by private surgeons.

Many private practitioners are actively involved in scientific organizations and companies that offer training programs to their younger colleagues.

As a private physician too, you can be one of the best physicians in the world.

# THE "OTHER" MEDICINE

Finally, I would like to talk to you about another type of medicine, which we call global medicine.

Although historically there have been physicians dedicated to the needs of our very poor and forgotten fellow humans around the world (who doesn't remember Dr. Albert Schweitzer?), so-called global medicine has only begun to develop in recent years. The largest American universities and hospitals now all have departments of global health and global surgery.

Recently, efforts have been made to coordinate many of these departments and organizations that serve the medical needs of poor people. The Global Alliance for Surgical, Obstetric, Trauma and Anaesthesia Care

(The G4 Alliance) is one of these efforts. Involving 80 organizations from 160 countries, the G4 Alliance is working to raise awareness of the world's modern-day needs for safety in surgery and childbirth, and for better treatment of the multi-injured. These needs are, in some countries, greater than the needs for clean water, infection control and HIV-specific infections.

I was recently in a large university hospital in an economically developing country in Africa. It's a big hospital, and lots of poor patients, with their relatives, all were gathered in and around the hospital. In the Department of Surgery they very politely tried every day, from morning to night, to serve the hundreds of patients who were gathered in the outpatient clinics. They lacked the means to perform even a simple laparoscopic gallbladder removal, yet they performed most "open" surgical procedures with self-sacrifice.

The surgeons I met had the same ambitions and the same dreams for their personal advancement and further training as all their colleagues in developed countries. They cared for their patients, their students, and their specialist new colleagues just like an academic surgeon would in the United States and Europe.

Despite the huge shortages in technical, hospital and pharmaceutical equipment, they experienced the joy of helping the sick. They felt the deep satisfaction that all physicians have who meet the needs of their patients no matter where in the world they may be living and working.

I know several academically very well trained physicians who decided to practice this "other" medicine. They all talk about a special joy and sense of fulfillment that they never knew in the big hospitals in Europe and the United States where they worked before going to the hospitals in Africa.

If your heart skips a beat at such a prospect, why not try it? Most prestigious universities and medical schools in the world have developed global health departments where you can easily get information on where and how you can experience the joys and challenges of this "other" medicine.

Begin by taking part in an existing program in Ethiopia, Tanzania or Mongolia, for example, for a short period of one or two months. If you like it, stay on for longer. You may end up devoting yourself to this "other" medicine that offers different joys than the ones you will experience at a university, or a public or private hospital in your economically developed country.

# THE DANGER OF BURNOUT

In recent years, at an increasingly growing rate, physicians of all ages are experiencing burnout syndrome. The definition of burnout includes a sense of emotional exhaustion, a sense of alienation, and a reduction in one's professional efficacy.

According to recent studies in both the United States and the UK, burnout affects more than 50% of physicians in all specialties. In fact, according to an article published in *The Lancet*, this syndrome is showing an alarming increase among medical students and specialist physicians. Burnout increases the risk of cardiovascular disease, reduces life expectancy, disrupts interpersonal relations, and can lead to alcoholism, depression and suicide. In fact, The Physicians

Foundation recently launched a campaign to help raise greater awareness about the suicide epidemic among physicians. "One physician commits suicide every day, the highest suicide rate of any profession and more than twice that of the general population," according to the president of The Physicians Foundation.

This is not surprising given that the risk of burnout among physicians is significantly higher than the risk among all workers in the United States. In fact, according to a 2019 study in the Mayo Clinic Proceedings clinical journal, physicians are the least satisfied with their work-life integration. "Burnout in medicine right now is really an entire-profession problem," noted Professor Colin West of the Mayo Clinic." There's really no age group, career stage, gender or specialty that's immune from these issues," he stated. Although a recent study among 15,000 physicians found that the age between 40 and 54 is the most dangerous and most common for developing burnout syndrome, large percentages were also found among medical students and young physicians, as well as among older, mature and "successful" physicians.

There are many reasons for the psychological exhaustion of physicians (i.e., burnout syndrome), such as excessive time spent on red tape; not enough time spent on the physician-patient relationship, which is constantly being regulated by hospitals and insurance companies; and the steady decline of physicians' fees. Another serious cause of burnout syndrome among physicians, especially in certain specialties, is the increase in lawsuits for actual or alleged medical errors and complications. This ever-increasing legal action against physicians is causing them either to suffer emotional exhaustion or to turn to defensive medicine, in the event that they continue their careers. Many either stop practicing medicine altogether or change their specialty. Studies have shown that burned out physicians, who, as we have seen, now make up more than 50% of all physicians, lose their original love of the profession and don't wish for their children to follow in their footsteps.

In the next chapters I would like to share with you my thoughts on how you can prevent the very real danger of burnout and how to keep alive the love of medicine throughout your lives.

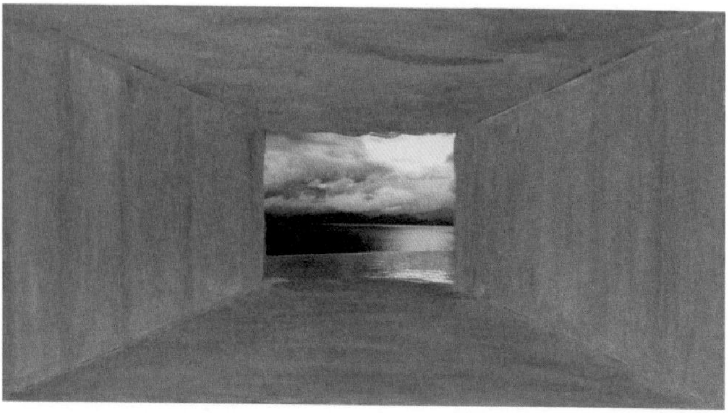

# FIND TIME

## For Yourself

The reality is that long before we even succeed in being accepted to medical school, we learn that it is a "bad thing" to have time to ourselves. The necessary tutorials to enter the medical school might have forced you to stop any extracurricular activities in sports, music, literature, or volunteering that you may have been involved in.

As a successful physician, your days and nights are dedicated to the sole purpose of getting into medical school and graduating with honors.

As a resident as well as practicing physician, you have been taught, like a hamster, to keep running on the wheel and never stop. Worst of all, you have been conditioned to think that this path will lead you to become the best physician for your patients and for society.

At this point I don't need to explain why this "good doctor" is already weary, he's burned out, he's lost his initial love of medicine, and he himself is in danger, as is his next patient.

We may be the "good doctor" for others but the worst for ourselves.

Which is why, at whatever stage of your career you might be (students, interns, residents, specialists, program directors, professors and even retirees), you must immediately put a stop to this vicious cycle of dedicating all your time to medicine, and to make sure you find time for yourself.

Here is some practical advice:

1. Start exercising regularly. Not every day, but certainly 3–4 times a week, go jogging outside, in the gym or on your treadmill at home, for half an

hour. For the remaining half an hour lift weights, do push-ups, and use TRX straps, thus doing a full hour of aerobic and non-aerobic exercise. On the weekends go for a hike in the countryside or do some light mountain climbing.

2. Rediscover any hobby you used to have: start those piano or guitar lessons you stopped years ago. Or take up a new hobby that you've never tried before. I suggest you buy some large canvases, tubes of acrylic paint and several paintbrushes. You won't believe how quickly you'll turn into an avid painter. And since you can't really go wrong with painting (especially the abstract kind), the mental relaxation it offers will be such that you won't want your spare time to end. You'll become completely engrossed, and then as soon as you finish your first painting, you'll be eager to start the second one.

3. Push yourself so that one day a week you attend a play, an opera, a lecture, a literary evening, a history presentation—anything other than medicine. Thanks to your cell phone, in just a few seconds you can get information about so many events that can give you deep joy and satisfy your

mind. Just think back to the elation you felt last time you attended a wonderful play, a concert, or a lecture. You deserve to relive many such pleasures.

4. Try for short periods each day to withdraw and clear your mind of its contents of that moment. Mindfulness is the modern-day directive for reducing daily stress: mindfulness means to be fully present, aware of where we are and what we're doing. Another similar term is meditation. You've probably heard of yoga, of the spiritual teacher who is called a guru, or of mantras—the syllables or group of words that are systematically recited (*japa*) while the speaker focuses his or her mind on their mystical meaning. Other alternatives, such as my own practice of the Greek Orthodox tradition, provide similar benefits. Any form of prayer, meditation or mindfulness will help us to rediscover the true joy of life. What is most important is that each person maintains inner spiritual balance, which is so necessary in dealing with our daily reality.

## For Your Partner

It's common knowledge that choosing the right partner is the key to a happy life. Especially for a physician, the right criteria for your initial choice of partner will seal your future happiness or misery. Criteria such as the financial or social status of your future spouse's family will lead to future problems, since the new medical student or the new physician will soon need neither financial support nor status. Choosing a partner based on mutual love and respect for each other's choices and desires eliminates the main force of resistance to life's difficulties and ensures the happiness of any physician in all phases of his or her medical career.

That's why it's necessary to find time—lots of time—to keep this relationship warm and meaningful. I will say it outright and I don't mind if you take it the wrong way: The physician who easily succumbs to the many opportunities our profession offers for extramarital affairs and relationships is a fool. You are also a fool if you don't give your life partner the time they deserve, the person who often is the one who "made" you a good scientist, a respected professor, a powerful executive, a successful physician. The most neglected patients are physicians' spouses. When you're ill, when you're going through an academic crisis, when you're burned out, the source of your strength to become well again is your partner, your spouse. It's good to bear that in mind through all the phases of your life.

## For Your Children

If children come into your life, you must find the time to be close to them from a very early age—from infancy and all through childhood—because that is when their minds and characters are shaped. For physicians, this prerequisite to raise children who will be happy and successful in their lives is a very difficult achievement.

For physicians who are trying to finish their specialty, to advance their academic career, or to succeed in their professional career, finding time for their children is indeed a great accomplishment, the fruits of which will be savored years later, when the children have grown up. Time spent with your children should be quality time, and that means taking a personal interest in each child, from reading bedtime stories to going on trips and playing sports together. Watching television with your children or telling them to go and play with their friends is not quality time. It's amazing how quickly children grow up and leave home to study abroad, to carve their own individual life path. These "tiring" hours that, as a new physician, you will spend in order to meet the needs of each of your young children will later become happy memories, and will have provided substantial support to the emotional and intellectual maturity of your child.

## For Your Colleagues and Friends

A recent study by the American Academy of Family Physicians (AAFP) across the United States of over 5,000 physicians of various specialties showed that 71% were happy and 59% were satisfied with their lives. "Happiness" did not mean that stress was lacking. Indeed, only 35% of physicians had more happiness than stress. It's just that stress doesn't necessarily mean lack of happiness or low life satisfaction—it's just part of the job.

More than 80% had positive relationships with their colleagues and the nursing staff, but only half of the physicians reported positive relationships with the hospital administration.

While your presence at the hospital facilitates your interpersonal relationships with other physicians and the nursing staff, keeping the friends you had at school, at university, and throughout your internship and residency requires more effort; it requires finding time for your old and new friends.

Your colleagues and friends will be the ones who will stand by you when the modern-day wave of lawsuits hits you for alleged "medical errors or omissions."

Studies have shown that 75% to 99% of physicians of all specialties will necessarily feel the threat of litigation during their career. "Malpractice is at the top of the list of major stressors for most physicians," says Dr. Charles M. Balch, a professor of surgery at the University of Texas, in a relevant study. "It's right up there with financial distress, serious work-home conflicts, and life-and-death circumstances." A study by the American College of Surgeons, which involved 7,000 surgeons, found that one in four were already in the middle of such a lawsuit. These surgeons had feelings of emotional exhaustion, depression, frustration with their careers, and suicidal thoughts. This negative experience leads 42% of physicians to limit their professional activity, to not undertake operations with a high risk of complications, and to avoid patients with complex medical problems. These psychologically exhausted physicians do harm not only to themselves but also to their next patient.

An interesting finding of a study by the Boston Intraoperative Adverse Events Surgeons' Attitude (BISA) titled "The Surgeon as the Second Victim?" showed that during this dramatic experience, which included 66% anxiety, 60% guilt, and 42% shame, surgeons received the most support not from their family but from their colleagues. The physician, who up until then was a "God" and the center of admiration and gratitude of the patient and his relatives, suddenly becomes the most hated person by these very same people. The physician is the one who is to blame for every complication that occurred in the operating room or postoperatively. At this point the physician doesn't know where to turn. Their spouse and friends who are not physicians cannot understand the meaning of a postoperative complication or how awful the surgeon feels. The only ones who can offer support are their colleagues, and indeed their superiors and those who have themselves gone through this difficult situation that they are facing now. Both Harvard and Johns Hopkins' hospitals have developed peer support groups made up of volunteer colleagues for physicians who are experiencing these unpleasant situations.

Finding time to cultivate deep interpersonal relationships with your colleagues is, among other things, a security for serious crises that you will have to go through during your career as a physician.

# AN ALTERNATIVE PIECE OF ADVICE

So far I have given you advice from my experience as a "classical" physician: one of the tens of thousands—if not hundreds of thousands—of surgeons serving their patients around the world, and one of the thousands of surgeons who thinks he is "God" or "God's deputy." (As the old joke goes: What's the difference between a surgeon and God? God knows he's not a surgeon.)

Although I was lucky enough to be trained in the best hospitals in the United States and was fortunate to have a good wife and five good children—and despite the fact that I had the satisfaction of being a good surgeon and a good professor who was adored by most of his patients and students, despite all the honors and distinctions bestowed upon me by my colleagues from all over the world (I went as far as to become President of the International Society of Endocrine Surgeons), and despite my good health and relative financial comfort—I know deep down that there is another path that is much better than the one I followed.

I "saw" this other path in the life of a famous surgeon who recently died, Luke of Simferopol, also known as Saint Luke the Surgeon. I sensed the existence of this path at a monastery on Mount Athos when I met a Harvard professor who had left his chair to become a novice monk. I felt this other path from time to time as I talked with seemingly simple physicians, unknown to most, whose presence and smile alone rested your soul.

It is these physicians, these people with different life priorities to ours, that one should seek out and ask for advice.

In villages that not many people have heard of—such as Terrasson-Lavilledieu or Solan in France, Tolleshunt Knights in England, Ormylia in Greece, or Florence, Arizona and Pleasant Prairie, Wisconsin in the United States—you will find some of the most well kept secrets for young or older physicians who want to become acquainted with something different. Something higher and more essential to their lives.

My alternative piece of advice is:

Seek out and take the time to get to know this other view of medicine, a different path to the one most of us followed. Maybe then you will be not only the best physician in the world, but also the happiest physician in the world.

# AFTERWORD

Fotis Pavlatos

I had the good fortune of knowing the sum of Professor Dimitrios Linos' invaluable and creative contribution so far to the Science of Hippocrates' Art. And to deeply appreciate his important and multifaceted personality in the scientific and social sectors of our country and beyond its borders, always framed by the indestructible human values that we so desperately need. Especially today, amid the "sandstorm" of the globalization of everything and of high technology (the 4$^{th}$ Industrial Revolution), particularly in terms of the physician-patient relationship and in the important field of providing health services.

And there is no doubt that:
"Humanism in healthcare is characterized by a respectful and compassionate relationship between physicians

and their patients, based on the ideals of integrity, altruism, respect, empathy and service." (Arnold P. Gold Foundation)

Also, in today's "global society," as it is shaped by high technology and the globalization of the economy, and as it suffers from their negative impact on humanitarian, intellectual and social values, we physicians are called upon to play an essential role, by offering the invaluable, traditional humanitarian element of the Hippocratic Spirit. In this age of high technology, as the French biologist Jean Rostand wrote: "Science has made us gods before we were worthy of being men."

In this book, you will find valuable information regarding the physician-patient relationship amid the rapid developments of medical science, especially in the 21st century, which can be characterized as "the golden age of Medicine."

For over half a century as a clinical physician, teacher and researcher, I can say that I have witnessed the "transformation" of medical science. The changes that have taken place in its progress and development, especially in the fields of high technology, techno-and bio-medicine, are truly impressive and in some cases border on the miraculous. At the same time, however, I experienced changes on an international scale regarding the image of health professionals, who went from being knight saviors to so-called health providers.

The evolution of medical science—with its consequent transformation of the image of the physician, disruption of the physician-patient relationship, and loss of medical credibility—combine to produce the "Hippocratic Insufficiency Syndrome," as I have described it.

And yet, in the Hippocratic view, the patient must be treated as a human being in his or her entirety and the treatment must be directed not only to the body but also to the soul. Since then, this view has been the ideal framework for the physician-patient relationship, which nowadays, 2,500 years after Hippocrates, must be embraced by every health therapist, applying the spirit of—as defined by the global medical community—holistic therapy.

And there is no doubt that health occupies the first place in the five basic social issues faced by every country (health, social security, social welfare, social protection, and education). It is necessary, of course, that the medical training of our students and our young physicians be carried out, throughout the entirety of their education, within a broad humanitarian and social context, following the Hippocratic requirement of the humanitarian element and love of humanity. Our students must learn not only the mechanics of the body, but also the human nature that is inside the body.

Awareness of the physician-patient relationship, the psychosomatic and the social element, must constitute the philosophical substratum for the teaching of medicine. The physician is not only the scientist/healer of the soul and body, but must also behave as a human being among his or her suffering fellow human beings.

According to Professor Albert E. Gunn of the University of Texas-Houston Medical School, the problem lies in the selection of medical students. He believes that they should be chosen based more on their broader education in history, philosophy and literature, rather than just on basic technical science knowledge, as is common in entrance exams. It has been said that if you read two novels by Tolstoy, you'll learn much more than from psychology textbooks and psychiatric manuals.

There is no doubt that the teaching of the history of medicine, medical ethics, literature, and the social sciences and humanities in general is an essential aspect of medical education, dictated by the needs of modern society and crucial in shaping a physician's behavior in daily medical practice. The physician's human approach to the patient is essential, both in terms of the patient's cooperation and the enhancement of the humanitarian element in dealing with patients with difficult treatment problems, especially in cases of patients who do not recover.

Personally, I believe that in the physician-patient relationship, a valuable element is that of empathy, which develops not only thanks to medical education, but also as a result of the physician's overall learning, stance and outlook, in terms of his or her role as a health therapist.

And it is more than certain that high technology displaces the humanitarian element of close contact:

the physician-patient relationship. In this way, medical credibility suffers a crisis, at a time when progress in the fields of IT, bio-technology, the recent three-dimensional printing revolution, and of course the 4$^{th}$ industrial revolution (robotic medicine) and the science of medicine in general allows us to do much more than we could in the past for the prevention and treatment of serious illnesses. These "failures of success" according to Ernest M. Gruenberg, pose a major question: How can we meet the increased demands and expectations of our patients and society in general in an atmosphere of diminished respect for and weakened reputation of the medical personality?

The answer is clear: The cultivation of the humanitarian element, with an emphasis on humanitarian values and medical ethics, as determined by the spirit of the Hippocratic vocation, which is aimed at subordinating the "machine" to the physician rather than having the physician being part of the "machine" and simply a "health provider."

As I wrote in one of my poems, in this age of Techno-medicine:

> And the slave became—a machine, a master
> And man became—a master, a slave.
> Subordination to the Machine?
> Woe betide us!
> Don't you ever forget Man . . .

At this point, however, I would be remiss not to emphasize the fact that in Greece the medical corps boasts infinite examples of medical ethics, sacrifice, altruism and selflessness. But the way they are reported in the daily press and in the media does not always reflect the true heights of duty and dedication: the helicopters that crash carrying physicians who are doing their job, the frequent and exhausting hospital shifts, the countless hours in surgeries, the superhuman effort and anxiety in the ICU, the rural physician left to his own devices, the nighttime bugle calls, often calling to battle against death—all these things are the ties that bind us to our Hippocratic vocation. And beyond all these things, volunteering with Doctors of the World, Doctors Without Borders (Médecins Sans Frontières), and Heart Doctors, within and beyond our country's borders, even at war fronts, where everything is on fire. A daily struggle between life and death.

The problems of medical ethics are urgent today.

I had, I have, and I will always have a dream, a vision, to see this Global Neo-Hippocratic Torch Relay, to keep the undying flame, throughout the world, as it is written in a verse, in a poem of mine in English entitled: "The Torch."

> A torch procession across the earth
> (Addressed mainly to our younger colleagues)
> Now, that the time came
> Shall I light my torch
> In life's journey bright flame
> Will ever guide my thoughts.

Understanding all that was said previously about the shaping of the new physician's personality in today's age of high technology and super-intelligence through their stance, place and outlook on life, in terms of their role in the Hippocratic Art, we hand them the Torch of the Hippocratic Spirit, with these words:

> This torch
> Handed to you today
> Keep it aloft, undying

It is the symbol of knowledge and your guide
It is spirit and light.

**Professor Fotis Pavlatos** is considered one of the leading endocrinologists in the world. His work on inhibiting adrenal cortisol production following dexamethasone administration the night before remains, 50 years after its publication in *JAMA*, as one of the classic tests for diagnosing adrenal disease. The test is referred to internationally as the "Pavlatos test."

# ABOUT THE AUTHOR

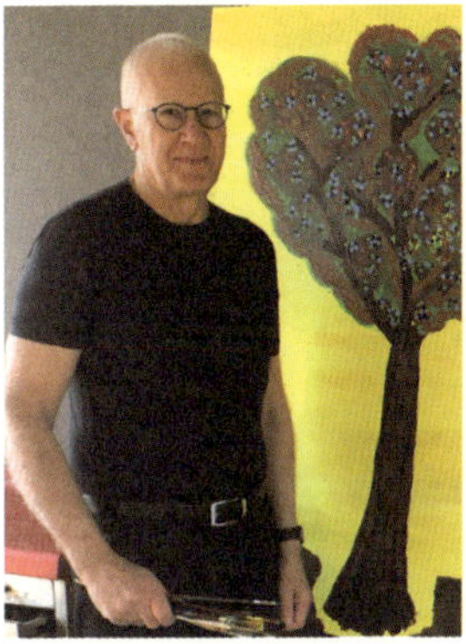

DIMITRIOS LINOS

Emeritus Professor of Surgery at the National and Kapodistrian University of Athens, and Lecturer in Surgery at Harvard University, Boston, MA.

He is an internationally acknowledged pioneer in Endocrine Surgery. As President of the International Association of Endocrine Surgeons (IAES) and Invited Professor at many international conferences, he has inducted thousands of surgeons in the USA, Europe, Asia and Africa in the modern treatment of thyroid, parathyroid and adrenal diseases. His experience in the surgical treatment of these conditions is currently probably the largest internationally. His Minimally Invasive Non-Endoscopic Thyroidectomy (MINET) technique has not only the best results regarding safety and the more radical thyroidectomy, but also the best aesthetic results.